DIABETES RENAL DIET COOKBOOK

Nourishing Meals for Kidney Health and Blood Sugar Control

ALBERT D MONK

Copyright © 2023 by Albert D Monk

Table of Contents

INTRODUCTION

Diabetes and chronic kidney disease often go hand in hand, forming a challenging health condition known as Diabetic Nephropathy. A crucial aspect of managing this dual burden lies in adopting a specialized dietary approach called the Diabetes Renal Diet.

Designed to preserve kidney function and control blood sugar levels, this diet empowers individuals with diabetes and renal complications to lead healthier lives.

The Diabetes Renal Diet focuses on a balanced and cautious intake of nutrients, especially sodium, potassium, phosphorus, and protein. It aims to alleviate the strain on the kidneys while keeping blood glucose levels in check.

By incorporating a variety of nutrient-dense foods, including whole grains, lean proteins, fresh fruits, and vegetables, individuals can ensure they receive essential nutrients without overburdening their kidneys.

Portion control and proper hydration play pivotal roles in this diet, preventing excessive waste build-up in the kidneys and maintaining adequate fluid balance. As diabetes and renal health can differ among individuals, healthcare professionals work closely with patients to customize their dietary plans, ensuring optimal management of both conditions.

CHAPTER 1

Understanding Diabetes and Kidney Health

Diabetes and kidney health are closely intertwined, and understanding their relationship is crucial for managing both conditions effectively. Diabetes is a chronic metabolic disorder characterized by high blood sugar levels, resulting from inadequate insulin production or the body's inability to effectively use insulin.

On the other hand, kidney health refers to the proper functioning of the kidneys, which play a vital role in filtering waste products and excess fluids from the blood.

The link between diabetes and kidney health is primarily due to the negative impact of consistently high blood sugar levels on the kidneys' delicate filtering units called nephrons. Over time, uncontrolled diabetes can cause damage to these nephrons, leading to a condition called diabetic kidney disease (DKD) or diabetic nephropathy.

Managing Diabetes with Kidney Disease

Managing diabetes with kidney disease is crucial to maintain overall health and prevent further complications. The coexistence of both conditions, known as diabetic kidney disease or diabetic nephropathy, requires a comprehensive approach to treatment. Some of the crucial points to consider are as follows:

1. Medical Team: Collaborate with a multidisciplinary medical team, including endocrinologists, nephrologists, dietitians, and educators, to create a tailored treatment plan.

2. Blood Glucose Control: Achieving and maintaining good blood sugar control is vital to slow the progression of kidney disease. Regularly monitor blood glucose levels and adjust insulin or medications as needed.

3. Blood Pressure Management: Control high blood pressure through lifestyle modifications, such as a low-sodium diet, regular exercise, and medication prescribed by the doctor. Maintaining a target blood pressure helps protect the kidneys.

4. Medication Review: Ensure all medications, including over-the-counter drugs and supplements, are kidney-friendly. Some medications may be harmful to the kidneys, so consult your medical team before starting any new medication.

5. Kidney-Friendly Diet: Adopt a kidney-friendly diet that is also suitable for diabetes management. Typically, this entails consuming less sodium, phosphorus, and potassium. Focus on whole grains, lean proteins, fruits, and vegetables.

6. Weight Management: Achieving and maintaining a healthy weight can positively impact both diabetes and kidney disease. Your medical team can help create a personalized weight management plan.

7. Regular Exercise: Engage in regular physical activity, as it can improve insulin sensitivity and promote overall health. Consult with your medical team to determine safe exercise options.

8. Avoid Smoking and Alcohol: Smoking and excessive alcohol consumption can further damage the kidneys and negatively affect diabetes management. Quit smoking and limit alcohol intake.

9. Medication Adherence: Take medications as prescribed and attend regular medical appointments. Adhering to your treatment plan is essential to manage both conditions effectively.

10. Blood Lipid Control: Keep cholesterol and triglyceride levels within a healthy range, as they can impact kidney and cardiovascular health.

11. Regular Kidney Function Monitoring: Regularly monitor kidney function through blood tests. Early detection of any decline in kidney function allows for timely intervention.

12. Education and Support: Learn about diabetes and kidney disease through education programs and support groups. Understanding both conditions empowers you to manage them effectively.

Remember, individual needs may vary, so always consult your medical team for personalized advice. By actively managing diabetes and kidney disease, you can enhance your quality of life and reduce the risk of complications.

Nutritional Guidelines for Diabetes and Kidney Patients

When managing diabetes and kidney disease, a well-balanced and tailored diet is crucial for maintaining blood sugar levels and kidney function. Here are some comprehensive nutritional guidelines to consider for individuals with both conditions:

1. Consult a Healthcare Professional: Before making any dietary changes, consult with a registered dietitian or healthcare professional familiar with diabetes and kidney disease. They can create a personalized plan that suits your specific health needs.

2. Manage Carbohydrate Intake: For diabetes control, monitor carbohydrate intake to regulate blood sugar levels. Choose complex carbohydrates like whole grains,

vegetables, and legumes instead of refined sugars and processed foods.

3. Control Sodium (Salt) Intake: Reducing sodium is essential for kidney health, as it helps manage blood pressure and fluid balance. Aim for less than 2,300 mg of sodium per day, or as per your healthcare provider's recommendation.

4. Limit Phosphorus and Potassium: For kidney patients, it's crucial to manage phosphorus and potassium levels in the blood. Foods high in phosphorus, such as dairy products and nuts, and those high in potassium, like bananas and potatoes, should be consumed in moderation.

5. Moderate Protein Intake: Balancing protein intake is important, as excessive protein consumption can strain the kidneys. Incorporate high-quality protein sources like lean meats, fish, poultry, and plant-based options.

6. Choose Healthy Fats: Opt for healthy fats like those found in avocados, nuts, seeds, and olive oil. Limit saturated fats and trans fats to promote heart health.

7. Stay Hydrated: Proper hydration is crucial for kidney function. Monitor fluid intake based on your doctor's recommendations, as excessive fluid retention can be harmful to the kidneys.

8. Monitor Blood Glucose Levels: Regularly check blood glucose levels and adjust your diet and medications accordingly to maintain stable blood sugar levels.

9. Spread Meals throughout the Day: Eating smaller, frequent meals can help manage blood sugar and prevent spikes in glucose levels.

10. Avoid Alcohol and Smoking: Both alcohol and smoking can worsen kidney function and diabetes complications, so it's best to avoid them altogether.

11. Consider Meal Planning: Creating meal plans can help you stay on track with your dietary goals, ensuring balanced nutrition and portion control.

12. Supplement with Caution: If needed, work with your healthcare provider to determine appropriate vitamin and mineral supplements, as some can interact with medications or impact kidney function.

Remember that individual dietary needs may vary, so always consult your healthcare team before making any significant changes to your diet. Regular monitoring and follow-ups are essential to assess progress and adjust the nutritional plan accordingly.

CHAPTER 2

Breakfast and Brunch Recipes

1. Spinach and Mushroom Egg White Omelette

Ingredients:

- Egg whites
- Spinach
- Mushrooms
- Salt
- Pepper
- Olive oil.

Instructions:

1. Whisk egg whites, sauté spinach and mushrooms in olive oil, add seasoned egg whites

2. Cook until set.

Prep Time: Approximately 15 minutes.

Nutritional Value (approx.):

- Calories: 150

- Protein: 15g
- Fat: 5g
- Carbohydrates: 7g
- Fiber: 2g

2. Breakfast Bowl of Quinoa with Berries and Almonds

Ingredients:

- Cooked quinoa
- Mixed berries
- Almonds, honey (optional)
- Greek yogurt (optional).

Instructions:

1. Mix cooked quinoa with berries and almonds

2. Drizzle honey and/or add Greek yogurt if desired.

Prep Time: Approximately 10 minutes (if quinoa is pre-cooked).

Nutritional Value (approx.):

- Calories: 350
- Protein: 10g

- Fat: 12g
- Carbohydrates: 45g
- Fiber: 8g

3. Greek Yogurt Parfait with Nuts and Fresh Fruit

Ingredients:

- Greek yogurt
- Mixed fresh fruit
- Nuts (e.g., almonds, walnuts)
- Honey (optional).

Instructions:

1. Layer Greek yogurt, fresh fruit, and nuts in a glass

2. Drizzle honey if desired.

Prep Time: Approximately 5 minutes.

Nutritional Value (approx.):

- Calories: 250
- Protein: 12g
- Fat: 10g
- Carbohydrates: 30g

- Fiber: 4g

4. Zucchini and Carrot Fritters with Greek Yogurt Dip

Ingredients:

- Zucchini
- Carrots
- Eggs
- Flour (all-purpose or almond flour)
- Baking powder
- Salt
- Pepper
- Greek yogurt
- Lemon juice
- Garlic.

Instructions:

1. Grate zucchini and carrots, mix with eggs, flour, baking powder, salt, and pepper.

2. Fry spoonfuls until golden.

3. Serve with Greek yogurt dip mixed with lemon juice and garlic.

Prep Time: Approximately 30 minutes.

Nutritional Value (approx.):

- Calories: 220
- Protein: 12g
- Fat: 6g
- Carbohydrates: 30g
- Fiber: 5g

5. Oatmeal with Chia Seeds and Cinnamon

Ingredients:

- Rolled oats
- Chia seeds
- Almond milk (or any milk of choice)
- Cinnamon
- Honey (optional)
- Fresh fruits (optional).

Instructions:

1. Cook oats with chia seeds and almond milk

2. Add cinnamon and honey for sweetness

3. Top with fresh fruits if desired.

Prep Time: Approximately 10 minutes.

Nutritional Value (approx.):

- Calories: 300
- Protein: 10g
- Fat: 8g
- Carbohydrates: 45g
- Fiber: 9g.

6. Breakfast Burrito with Whole Wheat Tortilla and Black Beans

Ingredients:

- Whole wheat tortilla
- Black beans
- Scrambled eggs
- Diced vegetables (e.g., bell peppers, onions)
- Salsa
- Avocado (optional).

Instructions:

1. Fill whole wheat tortilla with black beans, scrambled eggs, diced vegetables, salsa, and avocado if desired.

2. Roll into a burrito.

Prep Time: Approximately 20 minutes.

Nutritional Value (approx.):

- Calories: 400
- Protein: 15g
- Fat: 10g
- Carbohydrates: 55g
- Fiber: 12g.

7. Cottage Cheese Pancakes with Sugar-Free Syrup

Ingredients:

- Cottage cheese
- Eggs
- Oats
- Baking powder
- Vanilla extract
- Sugar-free syrup.

Instructions:

1. Blend cottage cheese, eggs, oats, baking powder, and vanilla extract.

2. Cook as pancakes and serve with sugar-free syrup.

Prep Time: Approximately 20 minutes.

Nutritional Value (approx.):

- Calories: 280
- Protein: 20g
- Fat: 10g
- Carbohydrates: 25g
- Fiber: 3g.

8. Avocado and Tomato Toast on Whole Grain Bread

Ingredients:

- Avocado
- Tomatoes
- Whole grain bread
- Lemon juice
- Salt
- Pepper
- Red pepper flakes (optional).

Instructions:

1. Mash avocado with lemon juice, spread on toasted whole grain bread

2. Top with sliced tomatoes

3. Season with salt, pepper, and red pepper flakes if desired.

Prep Time: Approximately 10 minutes.

Nutritional Value (approx.):

- Calories: 320
- Protein: 8g
- Fat: 15g
- Carbohydrates: 40g
- Fiber: 10g.

9. Veggie and Cheese Frittata with Egg Whites

Ingredients:

- Egg whites
- Mixed vegetables (e.g., bell peppers, spinach, onions)
- Shredded cheese (e.g., cheddar or feta)
- Salt
- Pepper.

Instructions:

1. Whisk egg whites, add mixed vegetables and shredded cheese

2. Season with salt and pepper. Bake until set.

Prep Time: Approximately 25 minutes.

Nutritional Value (approx.):

- Calories: 180
- Protein: 20g
- Fat: 8g
- Carbohydrates: 8g
- Fiber: 2g.

10. Smoothie with Spinach, Berries, and Almond Milk

Ingredients:

- Fresh spinach
- Mixed berries
- Almond milk
- Banana (optional)
- Chia seeds (optional).

Instructions:

1. Blend spinach, mixed berries, almond milk, and banana (if using) until smooth.

2. Add chia seeds for extra nutrients and fiber.

Prep Time: Approximately 5 minutes.

Nutritional Value (approx.):

- Calories: 200
- Protein: 5g
- Fat: 6g
- Carbohydrates: 35g
- Fiber: 8g.

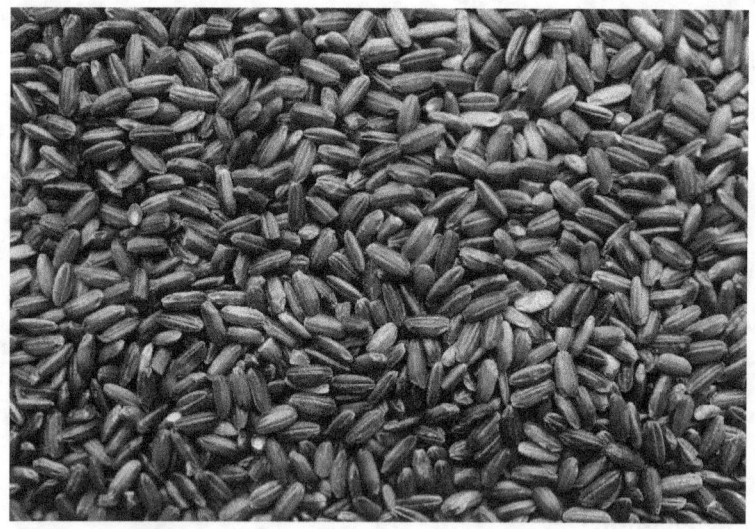

Brown Rice

CHAPTER 3

Appetizers and Snacks

11. Cucumber and Radish Salad with Lemon Vinaigrette

Ingredients:

- Cucumbers
- Radishes
- Lemon
- Olive oil
- Dijon mustard
- Honey
- Fresh dill
- Salt and pepper

Instructions:

1. Slice cucumbers and radishes thinly.

2. In a bowl, whisk lemon juice, olive oil, Dijon mustard, honey, dill, salt, and pepper to make the vinaigrette.

3. Toss the sliced cucumbers and radishes with the lemon vinaigrette.

4. Serve chilled.

Prep Time: 15 minutes

Nutritional Value:

- Calories: 80
- Carbs: 10g
- Fat: 4g
- Protein: 2g
- Fiber: 2g

12. Baked Sweet Potato Fries with Low-Sodium Seasoning

Ingredients:

- Sweet potatoes
- Olive oil
- Low-sodium seasoning (e.g., paprika, garlic powder, onion powder)
- Salt and pepper

Instructions:

1. Put parchment paper on a baking pan and preheat the oven to 425°F (220°C).

2. Cut sweet potatoes into thin strips.

3. In a bowl, toss sweet potato strips with olive oil and low-sodium seasoning.

4. Spread the seasoned sweet potatoes in a single layer on the baking sheet.

Bake for 20-25 minutes, or until crispy.

Prep. Time: 10 minutes
Baking Time: 20-25 minutes

Nutritional Value:

- Calories: 120
- Carbs: 25g
- Fat: 2g
- Protein: 2g
- Fiber: 4g

13. Edamame Hummus with Fresh Vegetables

Ingredients:

- Edamame beans (shelled)
- Tahini

- Lemon juice
- Garlic
- Olive oil
- Water
- Salt and pepper
- Assorted fresh vegetables for dipping (carrots, cucumbers, bell peppers, etc.)

Instructions:

1. Boil or steam edamame beans until tender.

2. In a food processor, blend edamame beans, tahini, lemon juice, garlic, olive oil, and water until smooth.

3. Season with salt and pepper to taste.

4. Serve with fresh vegetable slices for dipping.

Prep. Time: 15 minutes
Cooking Time: 5 minutes

Nutritional Value:

- Calories: 100
- Carbs: 6g
- Fat: 7g
- Protein: 5g
- Fiber: 3g

14. Tuna Lettuce Wraps with Avocado Slices

Ingredients:

- Canned tuna (in water or olive oil)
- Lettuce leaves (e.g., romaine or butter lettuce)
- Avocado
- Red onion (optional)
- Lemon juice
- Olive oil
- Salt and pepper

Instructions:

1. Drain the canned tuna and place it in a bowl.

2. Dice the avocado and red onion (if using) and add them to the tuna.

3. Drizzle lemon juice and olive oil over the mixture and season with salt and pepper.

4. Mix everything gently until well combined.

5. Spoon the tuna mixture onto lettuce leaves and wrap them up to form wraps.

Prep Time: 10 minutes

Nutritional Value:

- Calories: 200
- Carbs: 10g
- Fat: 10g
- Protein: 20g
- Fiber: 5g

15. Baked Parmesan Zucchini Chips: Ingredients

- Zucchini
- Grated Parmesan cheese
- Breadcrumbs
- Olive oil
- Garlic powder
- Salt and pepper

Instructions:

1. A baking sheet should be lined with parchment paper and the oven should be preheated to 425°F (220°C).

2. Slice zucchini into thin rounds.

3. In a bowl, mix grated Parmesan cheese, breadcrumbs, garlic powder, salt, and pepper.

4. Dip each zucchini slice in olive oil, then coat with the Parmesan mixture.

5. Place the coated zucchini slices on the baking sheet in a single layer.

6. Bake for 15-20 minutes or until golden and crispy.

Prep. Time: 15 minutes
Baking Time: 15-20 minutes

Nutritional Value:

- Calories: 120
- Carbs: 8g
- Fat: 7g
- Protein: 6g
- Fiber: 2g

16. Deviled Eggs with Greek Yogurt and Mustard

Ingredients:

- Hard-boiled eggs

- Greek yogurt
- Dijon mustard
- Lemon juice
- Paprika
- Salt and pepper
- Fresh parsley (optional, for garnish)

Instructions:

1. Cut hard-boiled eggs in half lengthwise and remove the yolks.

2. In a bowl, mash the egg yolks with Greek yogurt, Dijon mustard, lemon juice, salt, and pepper until smooth.

3. The yolk mixture should be added again to the egg white halves.

4. Sprinkle with paprika and garnish with fresh parsley, if desired.

Prep Time: 10 minutes

Nutritional Value:

- Calories: 70
- Carbs: 1g
- Fat: 4g
- Protein: 6g

- Fiber: 0g

17. Roasted Chickpeas with Herbs and Spices

Ingredients:

- Canned chickpeas (garbanzo beans)
- Olive oil
- Ground cumin
- Paprika
- Garlic powder
- Salt and pepper
- Fresh herbs (e.g., parsley, cilantro) for garnish

Instructions:

1. Put parchment paper on a baking pan and preheat the oven to 400°F (200°C).

2. Rinse and drain the canned chickpeas, then pat them dry with a paper towel.

3. In a bowl, toss the chickpeas with olive oil, ground cumin, paprika, garlic powder, salt, and pepper until evenly coated.

4. Cover the baking pan with a single layer of the seasoned chickpeas.

5. The chickpeas should be crispy after roasting for 25 to 30 minutes, with intermittent shaking of the pan.

6. Garnish with fresh herbs before serving.

Prep Time: 10 minutes
Roasting Time: 25-30 minutes

Nutritional Value:

- Calories: 130
- Carbs: 15g
- Fat: 4g
- Protein: 6g
- Fiber: 5g

18. Stuffed Bell Peppers with Lean Ground Turkey

Ingredients:

- Bell peppers (assorted colors)
- Lean ground turkey
- Brown rice (cooked)
- Onion
- Garlic
- Tomato sauce
- Italian seasoning

- Salt and pepper
- Shredded mozzarella cheese (optional, for topping)

Instructions:

1. Preheat oven to 375°F (190°C) and prepare a baking dish.

2. Scoop off the seeds and membranes after removing the bell peppers' tops.

3. In a skillet, cook lean ground turkey with chopped onions and minced garlic until browned.

4. Stir in cooked brown rice, tomato sauce, Italian seasoning, salt, and pepper.

5. Stuff the bell peppers with the turkey and rice mixture.

6. Place the stuffed peppers in the baking dish and cover with foil.

7. Bake the peppers for 25–30 minutes, or until they are soft.

8. Optionally, remove the foil, sprinkle shredded mozzarella cheese on top, and bake for an additional 5 minutes until the cheese melts.

Prep. Time: 20 minutes
Cooking Time: 30 minutes

Nutritional Value:

- Calories: 300
- Carbs: 25g
- Fat: 10g
- Protein: 25g
- Fiber: 5g

19. Turkey and Vegetable Lettuce Wraps: Ingredients

- Lean ground turkey
- Onion
- Garlic
- Carrots
- Red bell pepper
- Hoisin sauce
- Soy sauce
- Sesame oil
- Lettuce leaves (e.g., iceberg or butter lettuce)
- Green onions (optional, for garnish)

Instructions:

1. In a skillet, cook lean ground turkey with chopped onions and minced garlic until cooked through.

2. Add diced carrots and red bell pepper to the skillet and cook until tender.

3. Stir in hoisin sauce, soy sauce, and a dash of sesame oil to add flavor.

4. Place lettuce leaves with the turkey and veggie mixture on top.

5. Garnish with sliced green onions if desired and serve the wraps.

Prep. Time: 15 minutes
Cooking Time: 15 minutes

Nutritional Value:

- Calories: 200
- Carbs: 10g
- Fat: 8g
- Protein: 20g
- Fiber: 2g

20. Baked Buffalo Cauliflower Bites with Yogurt Dip

Ingredients:

- Cauliflower florets
- Olive oil
- Hot sauce (preferably Buffalo sauce)
- Whole wheat flour
- Garlic powder
- Salt and pepper
- Plain yogurt
- Dried dill
- Lemon juice

Instructions:

1. Set a baking sheet on the counter and preheat the oven to 450°F (230°C).

2. In a bowl, toss cauliflower florets with olive oil and hot sauce until well coated.

3. In a separate bowl, mix whole wheat flour, garlic powder, salt, and pepper.

4. Dredge each cauliflower floret in the flour mixture until evenly coated and place them on the baking sheet.

5. Bake for 20-25 minutes or until the cauliflower is crispy and lightly browned.

6. For the yogurt dip, mix plain yogurt with dried dill and a squeeze of lemon juice.

7. Serve the baked buffalo cauliflower bites with the yogurt dip on the side.

Prep Time: 15 minutes
Baking Time: 20-25 minutes

Nutritional Value:

- Calories: 100
- Carbs: 12g
- Fat: 4g
- Protein: 5g
- Fiber: 4g

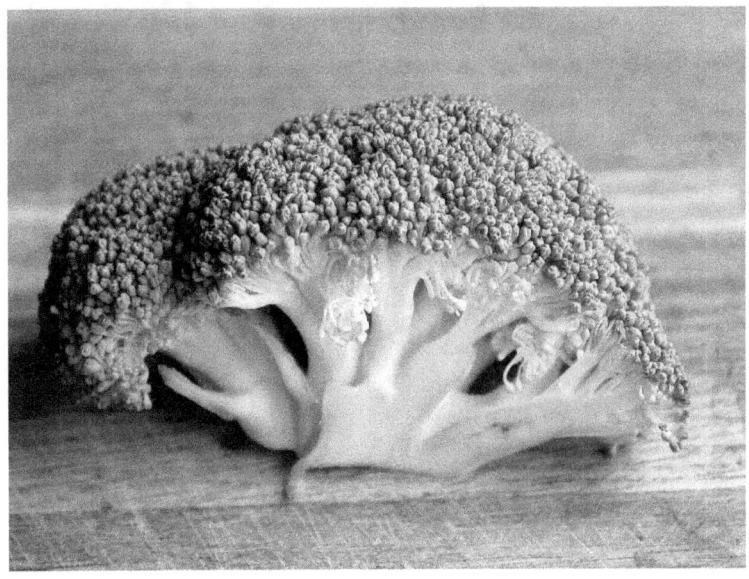

Broccoli

CHAPTER 4

Lunch and Dinner Entrees

21. Grilled Lemon Herb Salmon with Roasted Asparagus

Prep Time: 15 minutes

Ingredients:

- Salmon fillets
- Lemon slices
- Fresh herbs (rosemary, thyme, or parsley)
- Asparagus spears
- Olive oil
- Salt and pepper

Instructions:

1. Warm up the grill and give the grates a quick oiling.

2. Lemon juice, salt, and pepper should all be used to season the salmon fillets.

3. Add lemon slices and fresh herbs on the top.

4. Grill the salmon for 4-5 minutes per side or until cooked through.

5. Toss asparagus in olive oil, salt, and pepper. Roast in the oven at 400°F (200°C) for 10-12 minutes.

6. Serve the grilled salmon with roasted asparagus on the side.

Nutritional Values (per serving):

- Calories: 350
- Protein: 30g
- Carbohydrates: 10g
- Fat: 20g
- Fiber: 4g

22. Chicken Stir-Fry with Snap Peas and Brown Rice

Prep Time: 20 minutes

Ingredients:

- Chicken breast, thinly sliced
- Snap peas
- Bell peppers, sliced
- Onion, sliced

- Garlic, minced
- Ginger, grated
- Soy sauce
- Sesame oil
- Brown rice, cooked

Instructions:

1. In a wok or sizable pan, warm the sesame oil over medium-high heat.

2. Add the grated ginger and garlic, and cook for a minute until fragrant.

3. Add sliced chicken and cook until browned.

4. Stir in snap peas, bell peppers, and onion. Cook until vegetables are tender-crisp.

5. Stir-fry should be coated after adding soy sauce.

6. Serve the stir-fry over cooked brown rice.

Nutritional Values (per serving):

- Calories: 400
- Protein: 25g
- Carbohydrates: 40g
- Fat: 12g

- Fiber: 6g

23. Baked Cod with Lemon and Dill

Prep Time: 10 minutes

Ingredients:

- Cod fillets
- Lemon juice
- Fresh dill
- Garlic, minced
- Olive oil
- Salt and pepper

Instructions:

1. Preheat the oven to 375°F (190°C) and lightly grease a baking dish.

2. Place the cod fillets in the baking dish and season with salt and pepper.

3. In a small bowl, mix lemon juice, minced garlic, and chopped dill together.

4. Drizzle the lemon-dill mixture over the cod fillets.

5. Bake in the preheated oven for 15-20 minutes or until the fish is cooked through.

Nutritional Values (per serving):

- Calories: 200
- Protein: 30g
- Carbohydrates: 2g
- Fat: 8g
- Fiber: 0g

24. Turkey and Vegetable Skewers with Quinoa

Prep Time: 25 minutes

Ingredients:

- Turkey breast, cut into chunks
- Bell peppers, cut into chunks
- Cherry tomatoes
- Red onion, cut into chunks
- Zucchini, sliced
- Olive oil
- Lemon juice
- Italian seasoning
- Cooked quinoa

Instructions:

1. Preheat the grill or use a grill pan over medium heat.

2. Thread turkey chunks, bell peppers, cherry tomatoes, red onion, and zucchini onto skewers.

3. In a small bowl, whisk together olive oil, lemon juice, and Italian seasoning.

4. Apply the olive oil mixture to the skewers.

5. The skewers should be cooked through after 10 to 12 minutes of grilling, occasionally rotating them.

6. Serve the skewers over cooked quinoa.

Nutritional Values (per serving):

- Calories: 300
- Protein: 25g
- Carbohydrates: 20g
- Fat: 12g
- Fiber: 4g

25. Spinach and Mushroom Stuffed Chicken Breast

Prep Time: 30 minutes

Ingredients:

- Chicken breast
- Fresh spinach leaves
- Mushrooms, sliced
- Garlic, minced
- Mozzarella cheese, shredded
- Olive oil
- Salt and pepper

Instructions:

1. Preheat the oven to 375°F (190°C).

2. Butterfly the chicken breast to create a pocket for stuffing.

3. Sprinkle salt and pepper within the pocket.

4. In a pan, sauté garlic, mushrooms, and spinach until wilted.

5. Stuff the chicken breast with the sautéed mixture and shredded mozzarella.

6. Secure the pocket with toothpicks.

7. Bake in the preheated oven for 25-30 minutes or until chicken is cooked through.

Nutritional Values (per serving):

- Calories: 320
- Protein: 35g
- Carbohydrates: 5g
- Fat: 15g
- Fiber: 2g

26. Baked Eggplant Parmesan with Marinara Sauce

Prep Time: 40 minutes

Ingredients:

- Eggplant, sliced
- Egg
- Breadcrumbs
- Parmesan cheese, grated
- Mozzarella cheese, shredded
- Marinara sauce
- Fresh basil leaves
- Olive oil
- Salt and pepper

Instructions:

1. Preheat the oven to 400°F (200°C) and lightly grease a baking dish.

2. Dip eggplant slices in beaten egg, then coat with breadcrumbs mixed with grated Parmesan.

3. Lay the coated eggplant slices on the baking dish and drizzle with olive oil.

4. Bake for about 20-25 minutes or until the eggplant is tender and crispy.

5. Layer the baked eggplant slices with marinara sauce, shredded mozzarella, and fresh basil leaves.

6. When all the ingredients have been used, repeat the layering process, ending with a layer of mozzarella on top.

7. Bake for a further 15 minutes, or until the cheese is bubbling and melted.

Nutritional Values (per serving):

- Calories: 280
- Protein: 12g
- Carbohydrates: 20g
- Fat: 16g

- Fiber: 6g

27. Quinoa and Black Bean Stuffed Peppers

Prep Time: 25 minutes

Ingredients:

- Bell peppers
- Cooked quinoa
- Black beans, drained and rinsed
- Diced tomatoes
- Onion, chopped
- Garlic, minced
- Cumin
- Chili powder
- Shredded cheddar cheese
- Fresh cilantro
- Olive oil
- Salt and pepper

Instructions:

1. Preheat the oven to 375°F (190°C) and lightly grease a baking dish.

2. The bell peppers' tops are cut off, and the seeds and membranes are taken out.

3. In a pan, sauté onion and garlic in olive oil until softened.

4. Add cooked quinoa, black beans, diced tomatoes, cumin, chili powder, salt, and pepper. Mix well.

5. Place the quinoa and black bean mixture inside the bell peppers.

6. Place the stuffed peppers in the baking dish, cover with foil, and bake for 20-25 minutes.

7. Remove the foil, sprinkle shredded cheddar on top of the peppers, and bake for an additional 5 minutes or until the cheese is melted.

8. Garnish with fresh cilantro before serving.

Nutritional Values (per serving):

- Calories: 320
- Protein: 14g
- Carbohydrates: 45g
- Fat: 10g
- Fiber: 12g

28. Shrimp and Broccoli Stir-Fry with Brown Rice

Prep Time: 20 minutes

Ingredients:

- Shrimp, peeled and deveined
- Broccoli florets
- Bell peppers, sliced
- Carrots, sliced
- Garlic, minced
- Ginger, grated
- Soy sauce
- Sesame oil
- Brown rice, cooked

Instructions:

1. In a wok or large pan, heat sesame oil over medium-high heat.

2. Add the grated ginger and garlic, and cook for a minute until fragrant.

3. Stir in shrimp and cook until they turn pink and are fully cooked.

4. Add broccoli florets, sliced bell peppers, and carrots. Stir-fry until vegetables are tender-crisp.

5. Stir-fry should be coated with soy sauce after adding it.

6. Serve the shrimp and broccoli stir-fry over cooked brown rice.

Nutritional Values (per serving):

- Calories: 350
- Protein: 25g
- Carbohydrates: 45g
- Fat: 8g
- Fiber: 6g

29. Lemon Garlic Chicken with Steamed Green Beans

Prep Time: 30 minutes

Ingredients:

- Chicken thighs or breasts
- Lemon juice
- Garlic, minced
- Fresh thyme or rosemary
- Olive oil

- Salt and pepper
- Green beans, trimmed

Instructions:

1. Preheat the oven to 375°F (190°C).

2. In a bowl, mix lemon juice, minced garlic, chopped thyme or rosemary, olive oil, salt, and pepper.

3. Marinate the chicken in the lemon garlic mixture for at least 15 minutes.

4. Heat a skillet over medium-high heat and sear the chicken on both sides until golden brown.

5. Transfer the chicken to a baking dish and roast in the preheated oven for about 20-25 minutes or until fully cooked.

6. While the chicken is roasting, steam the green beans until tender-crisp.

7. Serve the lemon garlic chicken with steamed green beans on the side.

Nutritional Values (per serving):

- Calories: 320

- Protein: 30g
- Carbohydrates: 10g
- Fat: 18g
- Fiber: 4g

30. Spaghetti Squash with Turkey Bolognese Sauce

Prep Time: 1 hour

Ingredients:

- Spaghetti squash
- Ground turkey
- Onion, chopped
- Garlic, minced
- Crushed tomatoes
- Tomato paste
- Fresh basil leaves
- Olive oil
- Salt and pepper
- Grated Parmesan cheese (optional)

Instructions:

1. Preheat the oven to 400°F (200°C).

2. Cut the spaghetti squash in half lengthwise to remove the seeds.

3. Drizzle olive oil over the cut side of the squash and season with salt and pepper.

4. Place the squash halves cut-side down on a baking sheet and roast in the oven for 35-40 minutes or until the flesh is tender and easily scraped with a fork to form "spaghetti."

5. In a pan, sauté onion and garlic in olive oil until softened.

6. Add ground turkey and cook until browned and fully cooked.

7. Stir in crushed tomatoes, tomato paste, chopped fresh basil, salt, and pepper. Simmer for 15-20 minutes to let the flavors meld.

8. Once the squash is cooked, use a fork to scrape out the "spaghetti" strands into a serving bowl.

9. Top the spaghetti squash with the turkey Bolognese sauce and sprinkle with grated Parmesan cheese if desired.

Nutritional Values (per serving):

- Calories: 350
- Protein: 22g

- Carbohydrates: 30g
- Fat: 16g
- Fiber: 8g

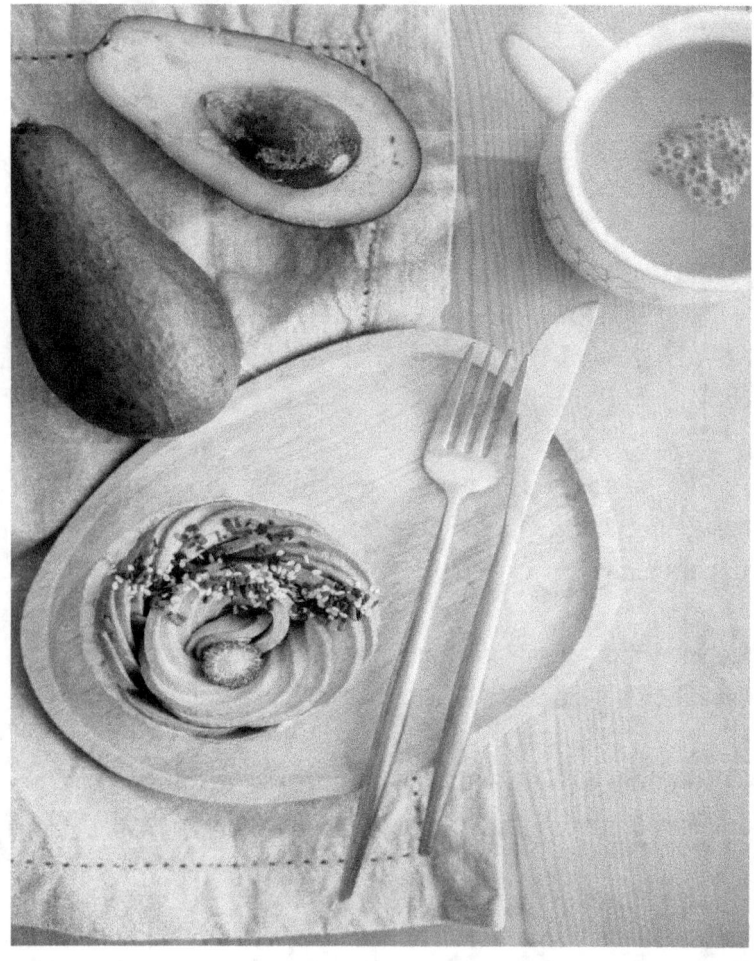

Avocado

CHAPTER 5

Sides and Salads

31. Roasted Brussels Sprouts with Balsamic Glaze

Prep time: 10 minutes

Ingredients:

- Brussels sprouts
- Olive oil
- Balsamic vinegar
- Salt and pepper

Instructions:

1. Preheat the oven to 400°F (200°C).

2. Trim and halve the Brussels sprouts.

3. Season with salt, pepper, and olive oil.

4. Spread them on a baking sheet and roast for 20-25 minutes until golden and tender.

5. Drizzle with balsamic glaze before serving.

Nutritional values (per serving):

- Calories: 120
- Fat: 6g
- Carbs: 14g
- Protein: 4g

32. Cucumber and Tomato Salad with Feta Cheese

Prep time: 15 minutes

Ingredients:

- Cucumbers
- Tomatoes
- Red onion
- Feta cheese
- Olive oil
- Lemon juice
- Fresh parsley
- Salt and pepper

Instructions:

1. Slice the cucumbers, tomatoes, and red onion.

2. Crumble the feta cheese on top.

3. In a separate bowl, whisk together olive oil, lemon juice, salt, and pepper for the dressing.

4. Toss the salad gently after adding the dressing.

5. Garnish with fresh parsley before serving.

Nutritional values (per serving):

- Calories: 160
- Fat: 10g
- Carbs: 12g
- Protein: 5g

33. Steamed Green Beans with Almonds

Prep time: 5 minutes

Ingredients:

- Green beans
- Sliced almonds
- Butter
- Lemon zest
- Salt and pepper

Instructions:

1. Steam the green beans until tender-crisp.

2. In a pan, toast the sliced almonds until lightly browned.

3. Toss the green beans with butter, lemon zest, salt, and pepper.

4. Sprinkle the toasted almonds over the top.

Nutritional values (per serving):

- Calories: 90
- Fat: 6g
- Carbs: 8g
- Protein: 3g

34. Kale and Cranberry Salad with Lemon Vinaigrette

Prep time: 20 minutes

Ingredients:

- Kale
- Dried cranberries
- Pecans
- Feta cheese
- Olive oil

- Lemon juice
- Honey
- Dijon mustard
- Salt and pepper

Instructions:

1. Wash and chop the kale leaves.

2. In a bowl, whisk together olive oil, lemon juice, honey, Dijon mustard, salt, and pepper for the dressing.

3. To soften the kale, gently massage the dressing into it.

4. Add the feta cheese crumbles, pecan halves, and dried cranberries.

5. Toss the salad before serving.

Nutritional values (per serving):

- Calories: 180
- Fat: 12g
- Carbs: 15g
- Protein: 5g

35. Grilled Vegetable Platter with Herb Seasoning

Prep time: 15 minutes

Ingredients:

- Assorted vegetables (bell peppers, zucchini, eggplant, etc.)
- Olive oil
- Fresh herbs (rosemary, thyme, oregano)
- Garlic powder
- Salt and pepper

Instructions:

1. Slice the vegetables and brush them with olive oil.

2. Sprinkle fresh herbs, garlic powder, salt, and pepper over the vegetables.

3. Vegetables should be grilled until soft and slightly browned.

4. Arrange them on a platter before serving.

Nutritional values (per serving):

- Calories: 100
- Fat: 6g
- Carbs: 10g
- Protein: 3g

36. Quinoa and Chickpea Salad with Lemon Dressing

Prep time: 25 minutes

Ingredients:

- Quinoa
- Chickpeas
- Cucumber
- Cherry tomatoes
- Red onion
- Fresh parsley
- Olive oil
- Lemon juice
- Garlic
- Salt and pepper

Instructions:

1. Quinoa should be prepared as directed on the package and then allowed to cool.

2. In a bowl, combine cooked quinoa, drained and rinsed chickpeas, diced cucumber, halved cherry tomatoes, and finely chopped red onion.

3. In a separate bowl, whisk together olive oil, lemon juice, minced garlic, salt, and pepper for the dressing.

4. Pour the dressing over the quinoa mixture and toss to combine.

5. Garnish with fresh parsley before serving.

Nutritional values (per serving):

- Calories: 220
- Fat: 8g
- Carbs: 30g
- Protein: 8g

37. Cauliflower Rice with Fresh Herbs

Prep time: 10 minutes

Ingredients:

- Cauliflower
- Olive oil
- Fresh herbs (parsley, mint, cilantro)

- Lemon zest
- Salt and pepper

Instructions:

1. In a food processor, pulse the cauliflower until it resembles rice after cutting it into florets.

2. In a pan, heat olive oil and sauté the cauliflower rice until tender.

3. Stir in fresh herbs, lemon zest, salt, and pepper before serving.

Nutritional values (per serving):

- Calories: 60
- Fat: 3g
- Carbs: 8g
- Protein: 3g

38. Greek Salad with Kalamata Olives and Feta Cheese

Prep time: 15 minutes

Ingredients:

- Cucumbers
- Tomatoes
- Red onion
- Kalamata olives
- Feta cheese
- Olive oil
- Red wine vinegar
- Dried oregano
- Salt and pepper

Instructions:

1. Dice the cucumbers, tomatoes, and red onion.

2. Toss them with Kalamata olives and crumbled feta cheese in a bowl.

3. In a separate bowl, whisk together olive oil, red wine vinegar, dried oregano, salt, and pepper for the dressing.

4. Pour the dressing over the salad and stir lightly before serving.

Nutritional values (per serving):

- Calories: 180
- Fat: 12g
- Carbs: 12g

- Protein: 5g

39. Steamed Broccoli with Garlic and Olive Oil

Prep time: 10 minutes

Ingredients:

- Broccoli florets
- Olive oil
- Minced garlic
- Lemon juice
- Salt and pepper

Instructions:

1. Steam the broccoli florets until tender-crisp.

2. Sauté minced garlic in olive oil in a skillet until fragrant.

3. Toss the steamed broccoli in the garlic oil mixture.

4. Add a splash of lemon juice, salt, and pepper before serving.

Nutritional values (per serving):

- Calories: 80
- Fat: 5g
- Carbs: 6g
- Protein: 4g

40. Spinach and Strawberry Salad with Balsamic Dressing

Prep time: 15 minutes

Ingredients:

- Baby spinach
- Fresh strawberries
- Goat cheese
- Candied pecans
- Balsamic vinegar
- Olive oil
- Honey
- Dijon mustard
- Salt and pepper

Instructions:

1. Wash and dry the baby spinach leaves.

2. Slice the fresh strawberries and crumble the goat cheese on top.

3. In a bowl, whisk together balsamic vinegar, olive oil, honey, Dijon mustard, salt, and pepper for the dressing.

4. Drizzle the dressing over the salad and top with candied pecans before serving.

Nutritional values (per serving):

- Calories: 220
- Fat: 14g
- Carbs: 18g
- Protein: 6g

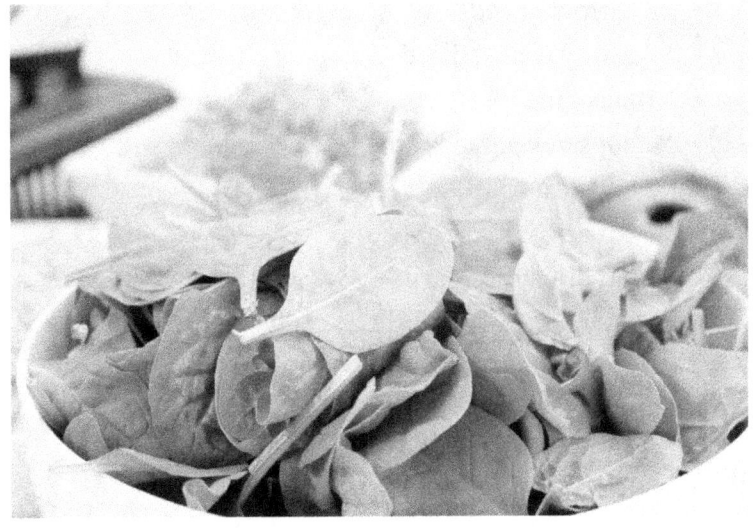

Spinach

CHAPTER 6

Soups and Stews

41. Lentil and Vegetable Soup with Herbs

Prep Time: 15 minutes

Ingredients:

- 1 cup dried lentils
- 1 onion, chopped
- 2 carrots, diced
- 2 celery stalks, diced
- 1 zucchini, diced
- 4 cups vegetable broth
- 2 cups water
- 1 tsp dried thyme
- 1 tsp dried rosemary
- Salt and pepper to taste

Instructions:

1. Sauté the chopped onion, carrots, and celery in a large pot until softened.

2. Add the lentils, vegetable broth, water, and dried herbs to the pot.

3. Bring to a boil, then reduce heat and let simmer for about 20-25 minutes or until lentils are tender.

4. Cook for 5 minutes more after adding the diced zucchini.

5. Season with salt and pepper to taste.

Nutritional Value (per serving):

- Calories: 240
- Protein: 15g
- Carbohydrates: 45g
- Fat: 1g
- Fiber: 12g
- Sodium: 500mg

42. Chicken and Vegetable Soup with Low-Sodium Broth

Prep Time: 20 minutes

Ingredients:

- 1 lb chicken breast, cooked and shredded
- 1 onion, chopped
- 2 carrots, sliced
- 2 celery stalks, sliced
- 4 cups low-sodium chicken broth

- 2 cups water
- 1 tsp dried thyme
- 1 bay leaf
- Salt and pepper to taste

Instructions:

1. Sauté the chopped onion, carrots, and celery until soft in a large pot.

2. Add the cooked and shredded chicken, low-sodium chicken broth, water, dried thyme, and bay leaf to the pot.

3. Bring to a simmer and let cook for about 15-20 minutes.

4. Season with salt and pepper to taste.

Nutritional Value (per serving):

- Calories: 180
- Protein: 25g
- Carbohydrates: 8g
- Fat: 4g
- Fiber: 2g
- Sodium: 300mg

43. Tomato and Basil Soup with Spinach

Prep Time: 10 minutes

Ingredients:

- 2 cans diced tomatoes
- 1 onion, chopped
- 3 cloves garlic, minced
- 4 cups vegetable broth
- 2 cups fresh spinach
- 1/4 cup fresh basil leaves
- 1 tbsp olive oil
- Salt and pepper to taste

Instructions:

1. In a large pot, sauté the chopped onion and minced garlic in olive oil until fragrant.

2. Add the diced tomatoes and vegetable broth to the pot.

3. Give the soup 10 minutes to simmer.

4. Stir in the fresh spinach and basil leaves until wilted.

5. Season with salt and pepper to taste.

Nutritional Value (per serving):

- Calories: 120

- Protein: 3g
- Carbohydrates: 15g
- Fat: 5g
- Fiber: 4g
- Sodium: 700mg

44. Minestrone Soup with Whole Wheat Pasta

Prep Time: 15 minutes

Ingredients:

- 1 cup whole wheat pasta, uncooked
- 1 onion, chopped
- 2 carrots, diced
- 2 celery stalks, diced
- 1 can diced tomatoes
- 1 can kidney beans, drained and rinsed
- 4 cups vegetable broth
- 2 cups water
- 1 tsp dried oregano
- 1 tsp dried basil
- Salt and pepper to taste

Instructions:

1. Cook the whole wheat pasta according to package instructions, then set aside.

2. Sauté the chopped onion, carrots, and celery in a large pot until softened.

3. Add the diced tomatoes, kidney beans, vegetable broth, water, dried oregano, and dried basil to the pot.

4. Give the soup 15-20 minutes to simmer.

5. Stir in the cooked whole wheat pasta.

6. Season with salt and pepper to taste.

Nutritional Value (per serving):

- Calories: 280
- Protein: 10g
- Carbohydrates: 50g
- Fat: 2g
- Fiber: 10g
- Sodium: 600mg

45. Vegetable and Bean Stew with Quinoa

Prep Time: 15 minutes

Ingredients:

- 1 cup quinoa, uncooked
- 1 onion, chopped
- 2 carrots, diced
- 2 celery stalks, diced
- 1 can black beans, drained and rinsed
- 1 can chickpeas, drained and rinsed
- 4 cups vegetable broth
- 2 cups water
- 1 tsp cumin
- 1 tsp paprika
- Salt and pepper to taste

Instructions:

1. Set aside the quinoa once it has been cooked according to the package directions.

2. Sauté the chopped onion, carrots, and celery in a large pot until soft.

3. Add the black beans, chickpeas, vegetable broth, water, cumin, and paprika to the pot.

4. Give the soup 10 minutes to simmer.

5. Stir in the cooked quinoa.

6. Season with salt and pepper to taste.

Nutritional Value (per serving):

- Calories: 320
- Protein: 12g
- Carbohydrates: 55g
- Fat: 5g
- Fiber: 12g
- Sodium: 700mg

46. Turkey and Kale Soup with Lemon Zest

Prep Time: 20 minutes

Ingredients:

- 1 lb ground turkey
- 1 onion, chopped
- 2 carrots, sliced
- 2 celery stalks, sliced
- 4 cups chicken broth
- 2 cups water
- 2 cups chopped kale
- Zest of 1 lemon
- Salt and pepper to taste

Instructions:

1. In a large pot, cook the ground turkey until browned, then set aside.

2. Sauté the chopped onion, carrots, and celery until softened.

3. Add the cooked ground turkey, chicken broth, water, and chopped kale to the pot.

4. Give the soup 15-20 minutes to simmer.

5. Stir in the lemon zest.

6. Season with salt and pepper to taste.

Nutritional Value (per serving):

- Calories: 250
- Protein: 20g
- Carbohydrates: 10g
- Fat: 10g
- Fiber: 3g
- Sodium: 600mg

47. Carrot and Ginger Soup with Greek Yogurt Swirl

Prep Time: 15 minutes

Ingredients:

- 1 lb carrots, chopped
- 1 onion, chopped
- 3 cloves garlic, minced
- 1 tbsp fresh ginger, grated
- 4 cups vegetable broth
- 2 cups water
- 1/2 cup Greek yogurt
- Salt and pepper to taste

Instructions:

1. The chopped onion and minced garlic should be cooked until aromatic in a big pot.

2. Add the chopped carrots, grated ginger, vegetable broth, and water to the pot.

3. Let the soup simmer for about 15-20 minutes or until carrots are tender.

4. Using an immersion blender or batches in a conventional blender, puree the soup.

5. Season with salt and pepper to taste.

6. Swirl in the Greek yogurt before serving.

Nutritional Value (per serving):

- Calories: 120
- Protein: 5g
- Carbohydrates: 20g
- Fat: 2g
- Fiber: 5g
- Sodium: 500mg

48. Chicken Tortilla Soup with Avocado Slices

Prep Time: 20 minutes

Ingredients:

- 1 lb chicken breast, cooked and shredded
- 1 onion, chopped
- 3 cloves garlic, minced
- 1 can diced tomatoes
- 4 cups chicken broth
- 2 cups water
- 1 tsp chili powder
- 1 tsp cumin
- Tortilla chips for serving
- Avocado slices for serving
- Fresh cilantro for garnish
- Lime wedges for serving

Instructions:

1. The chopped onion and minced garlic should be cooked until aromatic in a big pot.

2. Add the cooked and shredded chicken, diced tomatoes, chicken broth, water, chili powder, and cumin to the pot.

3. Give the soup 10 minutes to simmer.

4. Serve the soup topped with tortilla chips, avocado slices, fresh cilantro, and lime wedges.

Nutritional Value (per serving):

- Calories: 280
- Protein: 20g
- Carbohydrates: 20g
- Fat: 12g
- Fiber: 4g
- Sodium: 800mg

49. Split Pea and Ham Soup with Fresh Herbs

Prep Time: 15 minutes

Ingredients:

- 2 cups dried split peas
- 1 onion, chopped
- 2 carrots, diced
- 2 celery stalks, diced
- 2 cups diced ham
- 4 cups chicken broth
- 2 cups water
- 1 tsp dried thyme
- 1 tsp dried parsley
- Salt and pepper to taste

Instructions:

1. Rinse the dried split peas under cold water, then set aside.

2. The chopped celery, onion, and carrots should be sautéed until tender in a big pot.

3. Add the diced ham, chicken broth, water, dried thyme, and dried parsley to the pot.

4. Bring to a boil, then reduce heat and let simmer for about 30-40 minutes or until peas are tender.

5. Season with salt and pepper to taste.

Nutritional Value (per serving):

- Calories: 320

- Protein: 22g
- Carbohydrates: 50g
- Fat: 4g
- Fiber: 15g
- Sodium: 1000mg

50. Butternut Squash and Apple Soup with Cinnamon

Prep Time: 15 minutes

Ingredients:

- 1 butternut squash, peeled, seeded, and chopped
- 2 apples, peeled, cored, and chopped
- 1 onion, chopped
- 3 cloves garlic, minced
- 4 cups vegetable broth
- 2 cups water
- 1 tsp cinnamon
- 1/2 tsp nutmeg
- Salt and pepper to taste

Instructions:

1. The chopped onion and minced garlic should be cooked until aromatic in a big pot.

2. Add the chopped butternut squash, chopped apples, vegetable broth, and water to the pot.

3. Let the soup simmer for about 15-20 minutes or until squash and apples are tender.

4. Using an immersion blender or batches in a conventional blender, puree the soup.

5. Add to taste the cinnamon, nutmeg, salt, and pepper.

Nutritional Value (per serving):

- Calories: 140
- Protein: 2g
- Carbohydrates: 30g
- Fat: 1g
- Fiber: 6g
- Sodium: 500mg

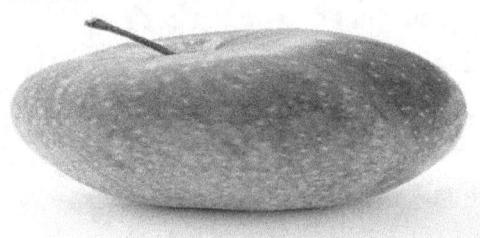

Apple

CHAPTER 7

Desserts and Sweet Treats:

51. Baked Apple Slices with Cinnamon and Walnuts

Prep time: 10 minutes

Ingredients:

- 3 apples, cored and thinly sliced
- 1 tablespoon cinnamon
- 1/4 cup chopped walnuts

Instructions:

1. Preheat the oven to 375°F (190°C).

2. In a mixing bowl, toss the apple slices with cinnamon until coated.

3. Spread the coated apple slices on a baking sheet lined with parchment paper.

4. Sprinkle chopped walnuts over the apple slices.

5. Bake in the preheated oven for 15-20 minutes or until the apples are tender and slightly golden.

Nutritional Value (per serving):

- Calories: 150
- Protein: 2g
- Carbohydrates: 25g
- Fat: 6g
- Fiber: 5g

52. Berry and Chia Seed Pudding with Coconut Milk

Prep time: 5 minutes (+ chilling time)

Ingredients:

- 1 cup mixed berries (strawberries, blueberries, raspberries)
- 1/4 cup chia seeds
- 1 cup coconut milk
- 1 tablespoon honey (optional)

Instructions:

1. In a jar or airtight container, combine the chia seeds and coconut milk. Stir well.

2. Add honey if desired, and mix until well combined.

3. Gently fold in the mixed berries.

4. Cover and refrigerate for at least 2 hours or overnight until the chia seeds have absorbed the liquid and the mixture thickens.

Nutritional Value (per serving):

- Calories: 250
- Protein: 5g
- Carbohydrates: 22g
- Fat: 17g
- Fiber: 12g

53. Greek Yogurt and Berry Popsicles

Prep time: 5 minutes (+ freezing time)

Ingredients:

- 1 cup Greek yogurt
- 1 cup mixed berries (blueberries, strawberries, blackberries)
- 2 tablespoons honey (optional)

Instructions:

1. In a blender, combine the Greek yogurt, mixed berries, and honey (if using).

2. Blend until smooth and well combined.

3. Pour the mixture into Popsicle molds.

4. Popsicle sticks should be inserted and frozen for at least 4 hours or until completely firm.

Nutritional Value (per serving):

- Calories: 120
- Protein: 6g
- Carbohydrates: 20g
- Fat: 1g
- Fiber: 3g

54. Banana and Walnut Muffins with Whole Wheat Flour

Prep time: 15 minutes

Ingredients:

- 2 ripe bananas, mashed
- 1/4 cup vegetable oil
- 1/2 cup honey or maple syrup

- 1 teaspoon vanilla extract
- 1 cup whole wheat flour
- 1 teaspoon baking powder
- 1/2 teaspoon baking soda
- 1/2 teaspoon cinnamon
- 1/4 teaspoon salt
- 1/2 cup chopped walnuts

Instructions:

1. Paper liners should be used to line a muffin pan and the oven should be preheated to 350°F (175°C).

2. In a large mixing bowl, combine the mashed bananas, vegetable oil, honey or maple syrup, and vanilla extract.

3. In a separate bowl, whisk together the whole wheat flour, baking powder, baking soda, cinnamon, and salt.

4. Add the dry ingredients gradually to the wet ingredients while stirring occasionally.

5. Fold in the chopped walnuts.

6. The batter should be divided among the muffin tins evenly.

7. Until a toothpick placed in the center of the cake comes out clean, bake for 18-20 minutes.

Nutritional Value (per muffin):

- Calories: 200
- Protein: 3g
- Carbohydrates: 25g
- Fat: 10g
- Fiber: 3g

55. Chocolate Avocado Pudding with Unsweetened Cocoa

Prep time: 10 minutes (+ chilling time)

Ingredients:

- 2 ripe avocados
- 1/4 cup unsweetened cocoa powder
- 1/4 cup honey or agave syrup
- 1 teaspoon vanilla extract
- Pinch of salt
- 1/4 cup almond milk (or any milk of your choice)

Instructions:

1. Remove the pits from the avocados by cutting them in half, then scoop the flesh into a food processor or blender.

2. Add the unsweetened cocoa powder, honey or agave syrup, vanilla extract, and a pinch of salt.

3. Blend until smooth and creamy, adding almond milk as needed to achieve your desired consistency.

4. Before serving, place the pudding in serving ware in the refrigerator for at least an hour.

Nutritional Value (per serving):

- Calories: 180
- Protein: 3g
- Carbohydrates: 21g
- Fat: 12g
- Fiber: 7g

56. Grilled Pineapple with Greek Yogurt Dip

Prep time: 15 minutes

Ingredients:

- 1 fresh pineapple, peeled and sliced
- 1 cup Greek yogurt
- 2 tablespoons honey
- 1 teaspoon vanilla extract

Instructions:

1. Preheat the grill to medium-high heat.

2. Grill the pineapple slices for 2-3 minutes per side or until grill marks appear.

3. To make the dip, combine the Greek yogurt, honey, and vanilla essence in a small bowl.

4. Serve the grilled pineapple with the Greek yogurt dip on the side.

Nutritional Value (per serving):

- Calories: 120
- Protein: 4g
- Carbohydrates: 28g
- Fat: 0.5g
- Fiber: 3g

57. Almond Flour Blueberry Bars with Stevia

Prep time: 10 minutes (+ baking time)

Ingredients:

- 1 1/2 cups almond flour
- 1/4 cup coconut oil, melted
- 2 tablespoons stevia (or any other natural sweetener)
- 1 teaspoon vanilla extract
- 1 cup fresh blueberries

Instructions:

1. Preheat the oven to 350°F (175°C) and grease a baking dish.

2. In a mixing bowl, combine the almond flour, melted coconut oil, stevia, and vanilla extract until crumbly.

3. Press two-thirds of the mixture into the bottom of the prepared baking dish.

4. Spread the fresh blueberries evenly over the crust.

5. Sprinkle the remaining almond flour mixture on top of the blueberries.

6. Bake for 25 to 30 minutes, or until the top is just beginning to turn brown.

7. Before cutting into bars, let the mixture cool fully.

Nutritional Value (per bar):

- Calories: 150
- Protein: 4g
- Carbohydrates: 10g
- Fat: 12g
- Fiber: 2g

58. Frozen Berry Sorbet with Lemon Zest

Prep time: 5 minutes (+ freezing time)

Ingredients:

- 2 cups mixed berries (strawberries, raspberries, blueberries)
- 1/4 cup honey or maple syrup
- 1 tablespoon lemon zest
- 1/4 cup water

Instructions:

1. In a blender, combine the mixed berries, honey or maple syrup, lemon zest, and water.

2. Blend until smooth and well combined.

3. Pour the mixture into a shallow dish or an ice cube tray.

4. Cover and freeze for a minimum of 3-4 hours, or until solid.

5. Once frozen, transfer the sorbet to a blender and blend again until smooth and creamy.

6. For a firmer texture, freeze for an additional 30 minutes before serving.

Nutritional Value (per serving):

- Calories: 100
- Protein: 1g
- Carbohydrates: 25g
- Fat: 0.5g
- Fiber: 4g

59. Coconut and Almond Energy Bites

Prep time: 15 minutes (+ chilling time)

Ingredients:

- 1 cup shredded coconut (unsweetened)
- 1/2 cup almond flour
- 1/4 cup almond butter
- 1/4 cup honey or agave syrup
- 1 teaspoon vanilla extract

- Pinch of salt

Instructions:

1. In a mixing bowl, combine the shredded coconut, almond flour, almond butter, honey or agave syrup, vanilla extract, and a pinch of salt.

2. Mix thoroughly until a sticky dough forms.

3. Roll the dough into bite-sized balls.

4. Place the energy bites on a parchment-lined tray and refrigerate for at least 30 minutes to firm up.

Nutritional Value (per energy bite):

- Calories: 80
- Protein: 2g
- Carbohydrates: 8g
- Fat: 5g
- Fiber: 1g

60. Cinnamon Baked Pear with Ricotta Cheese

Prep time: 10 minutes (+ baking time)

Ingredients:

- 2 ripe pears, halved and cored
- 1 tablespoon honey
- 1/2 teaspoon ground cinnamon
- 1/4 cup ricotta cheese

Instructions:

1. Preheat the oven to 375°F (190°C) and line a baking dish with parchment paper.

2. Place the pear halves in the baking dish, cut side up.

3. Drizzle honey over each pear half and sprinkle with ground cinnamon.

4. Bake in the preheated oven for 20-25 minutes or until the pears are tender.

5. Put a dollop of ricotta cheese over top and serve warm.

Nutritional Value (per serving):

- Calories: 120
- Protein: 2g
- Carbohydrates: 26g
- Fat: 2g
- Fiber: 5g

CHAPTER 8

Beverages and Smoothies:

61. Green Smoothie with Spinach, Avocado, and Cucumber

Prep Time: 5 minutes

Ingredients:

- 1 cup fresh spinach leaves
- 1/2 ripe avocado
- 1/2 cucumber, peeled and sliced
- 1 cup water or coconut water (unsweetened)
- Ice cubes (optional)

Instructions:

1. In a blender, combine spinach, avocado, cucumber, and water (or coconut water).

2. Blend until smooth and creamy.

3. Ice cubes may be added if preferred.

4. Blend again until thoroughly blended.

5. Pour into a glass and enjoy.

Nutritional Value (per serving):

- Calories: 120
- Carbohydrates: 8g
- Protein: 3g
- Fat: 10g
- Fiber: 5g

62. Watermelon and Mint Cooler

Prep Time: 10 minutes

Ingredients:

- 2 cups fresh watermelon, diced
- 6-8 fresh mint leaves
- 1 cup water
- Ice cubes

Instructions:

1. In a blender, combine watermelon, mint leaves, and water.

2. Blend until smooth.

3. Add ice cubes and blend again to chill the drink.

4. Pour into glasses and, if preferred, top with additional mint leaves.

Nutritional Value (per serving):

- Calories: 40
- Carbohydrates: 10g
- Protein: 1g
- Fat: 0g
- Fiber: 1g

63. Berry Blast Smoothie with Almond Milk

Prep Time: 5 minutes

Ingredients:

- 1 cup mixed berries (strawberries, blueberries, raspberries)
- 1 cup unsweetened almond milk
- 1 tablespoon honey or maple syrup (optional)
- Ice cubes

Instructions:

1. In a blender, combine mixed berries and almond milk.

2. Add honey or maple syrup if desired for greater sweetness.

3. Blend until smooth and creamy.

4. Blend again while adding ice cubes until thoroughly blended.

5. Pour into glasses and serve.

Nutritional Value (per serving):

- Calories: 150
- Carbohydrates: 20g
- Protein: 3g
- Fat: 6g
- Fiber: 4g

64. Cucumber and Lemon Infused Water

Prep Time: 2 minutes

Ingredients:

- 1/2 cucumber, sliced
- 1 lemon, sliced
- 4 cups water
- Ice cubes

Instructions:

1. In a pitcher, combine cucumber and lemon slices with water.

2. Refrigerate for at least 30 minutes to allow flavors to infuse.

3. Add ice cubes before serving.

Nutritional Value (per serving):

- Calories: 5
- Carbohydrates: 2g
- Protein: 0g
- Fat: 0g
- Fiber: 0g

65. Iced Hibiscus Tea with Stevia

Prep Time: 15 minutes

Ingredients:

- 2 tablespoons dried hibiscus flowers
- 4 cups water
- Stevia (or your preferred sweetener) to taste
- Ice cubes

Instructions:

1. In a saucepan, bring water to a boil and add hibiscus flowers.

2. Reduce heat and let it simmer for 10 minutes.

3. Remove from heat and let it cool.

4. Add stevia or your preferred sweetener to taste.

5. Refrigerate until chilled or add ice cubes before serving.

Nutritional Value (per serving):

- Calories: 0
- Carbohydrates: 0g
- Protein: 0g
- Fat: 0g
- Fiber: 0g

66. Pineapple and Ginger Smoothie with Coconut Water

Prep Time: 7 minutes

Ingredients:

- 1 cup fresh pineapple chunks
- 1-inch piece of fresh ginger, peeled and grated
- 1 cup coconut water (unsweetened)
- Ice cubes

Instructions:

1. In a blender, combine pineapple, grated ginger, and coconut water.

2. Blend until smooth and frothy.

3. Add ice cubes and blend again until well combined.

4. Pour into glasses and serve.

Nutritional Value (per serving):

- Calories: 80
- Carbohydrates: 20g
- Protein: 1g
- Fat: 0g
- Fiber: 2g

67. Avocado and Banana Smoothie with Unsweetened Almond Milk

Prep Time: 5 minutes

Ingredients:

- 1 ripe avocado
- 1 ripe banana
- 1 cup unsweetened almond milk
- 1 tablespoon honey or maple syrup (optional)
- Ice cubes

Instructions:

1. In a blender, combine avocado, banana, and almond milk.

2. Add honey or maple syrup if desired for added sweetness.

3. Blend until smooth and creamy.

4. Add ice cubes and blend again until well combined.

5. Pour into glasses and enjoy.

Nutritional Value (per serving):

- Calories: 250
- Carbohydrates: 30g
- Protein: 3g
- Fat: 15g
- Fiber: 8g

68. Blueberry and Kale Smoothie with Greek Yogurt

Prep Time: 6 minutes

Ingredients:

- 1 cup fresh blueberries
- 1 cup chopped kale leaves
- 1/2 cup Greek yogurt
- 1 cup water or milk (unsweetened)
- Ice cubes

Instructions:

1. In a blender, combine blueberries, kale, Greek yogurt, and water (or milk).

2. Blend until smooth and creamy.

3. Add ice cubes and blend again until well combined.

4. Pour into glasses and serve.

Nutritional Value (per serving):

- Calories: 160
- Carbohydrates: 20g

- Protein: 8g
- Fat: 5g
- Fiber: 5g

69. Mango and Lime Sparkling Water

Prep Time: 3 minutes

Ingredients:

- 1 cup fresh mango chunks
- Juice of 1 lime
- Sparkling water

Instructions:

1. In a blender, combine mango chunks and lime juice.

2. Blend until smooth.

3. Fill a glass with ice cubes and pour the mango-lime mixture over it.

4. Top up with sparkling water and stir gently.

Nutritional Value (per serving):

- Calories: 60

- Carbohydrates: 15g
- Protein: 1g
- Fat: 0g
- Fiber: 2g

70. Strawberry and Basil Lemonade

Prep Time: 8 minutes

Ingredients:

- 1 cup fresh strawberries, hulled
- 1/4 cup fresh basil leaves
- Juice of 2 lemons
- 4 cups water
- Honey or agave syrup to taste (optional)
- Ice cubes

Instructions:

1. In a blender, combine strawberries, basil leaves, lemon juice, and water.

2. Blend until well mixed.

3. Add honey or agave syrup if desired for added sweetness.

4. Refrigerate until chilled or add ice cubes before serving.

Nutritional Value (per serving):

- Calories: 40
- Carbohydrates: 10g
- Protein: 1g
- Fat: 0g
- Fiber: 2g

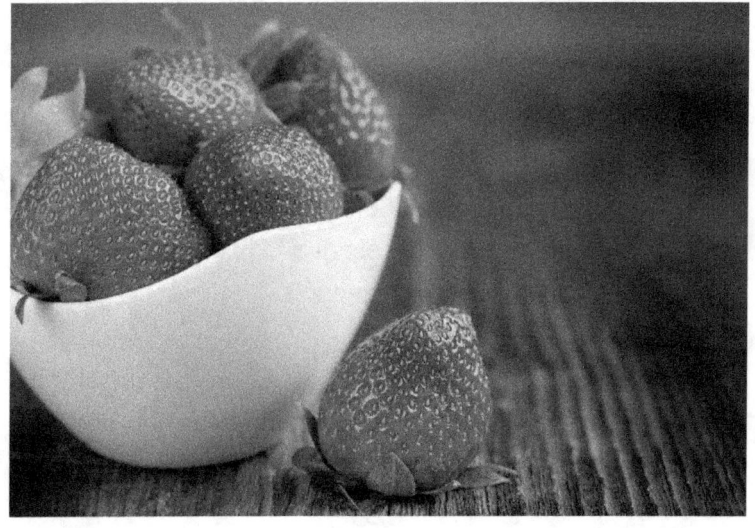

Strawberries

CHAPTER 9

Meal Planning and Prepping

Diabetes renal diet meal planning and prepping are essential for individuals who have both diabetes and kidney disease. The goal is to manage blood sugar levels and protect kidney function through a well-balanced and nutritious diet. Here are some general tips:

1. Understanding the Conditions:

- Diabetes: It is a metabolic disorder characterized by high blood glucose levels due to insulin resistance or insufficient insulin production.

- Renal (Kidney) Disease: Kidneys are responsible for filtering waste and excess fluids from the body. In renal disease, the kidneys may not function properly, leading to waste buildup.

2. Goals of Diabetes Renal Diet:

- Control Blood Sugar: Monitor and maintain stable blood glucose levels through balanced meal planning.

- Manage Kidney Function: Reduce the workload on the kidneys by moderating protein, phosphorus, and potassium intake.

- Control Blood Pressure: Limit sodium intake to help manage blood pressure.

3. Meal Planning Tips:

- Work with a Registered Dietitian: Seek guidance from a professional to create a personalized meal plan based on individual needs and medical history.

- Carbohydrates: Choose complex carbs with a low glycemic index to avoid rapid spikes in blood sugar.

- Protein: Moderation is key. Opt for high-quality, low-phosphorus sources like poultry, fish, and eggs.

- Fats: Emphasize healthy fats from sources like avocados, nuts, and olive oil.

- Sodium: Reduce salt intake by using herbs and spices for flavoring instead.

- Phosphorus and Potassium: Limit foods high in these minerals, such as dairy products, nuts, and bananas.

4. Prepping Diabetes Renal-Friendly Meals:

- Batch Cooking: Prepare larger quantities of renal-friendly meals and freeze them in individual portions for convenience.

- Food Safety: Practice proper food handling and storage to prevent contamination and spoilage.

- Portion Control: Measure portions to avoid overeating and to manage blood sugar levels effectively.

- Variety: Incorporate a diverse range of foods to ensure a balanced nutrient intake.

5. Meal Prepping Ideas:

- Grilled Chicken Breast with Roasted Vegetables

- Quinoa Salad with Cucumber, Tomato, and Feta Cheese

- Baked Salmon with Steamed Asparagus

- Stir-fried Tofu with Mixed Vegetables and Brown Rice

6. Hydration:

- Proper hydration is essential for kidney function. Choose water as the primary beverage and limit sugary drinks.

7. Monitoring and Adaptation:

- Regularly monitor blood sugar levels and kidney function with the guidance of healthcare professionals.

- Be open to adjustments in the meal plan as health conditions change.

It's essential to know that individual needs vary, so it's essential to work closely with healthcare professionals and a registered dietitian to create an effective and safe diabetes renal diet meal plan. By following these guidelines and planning meals carefully, individuals can improve their health and manage their conditions effectively.

Weekly Diabetic and Renal Meal Plans

Monday:

- Breakfast: Scrambled eggs with spinach and tomatoes

- Snack: Sliced cucumber with hummus

- Lunch: Grilled chicken salad with mixed greens and a vinaigrette dressing

- Snack: Greek yogurt with berries

- Dinner: Baked salmon with steamed asparagus and quinoa

Tuesday:

- Breakfast: Overnight oats with almond milk, chia seeds, and sliced peaches

- Snack: Carrot sticks with a small handful of almonds

- Lunch: Turkey and avocado wrap with whole-grain tortilla

- Snack: Cottage cheese with pineapple chunks

- Dinner: Stir-fried tofu with broccoli and brown rice

Wednesday:

- Breakfast: Smoothie with spinach, banana, unsweetened almond milk, and a dash of cinnamon

- Snack: Celery sticks with peanut butter

- Lunch: Lentil soup with a side of mixed vegetables

- Snack: Apple slices with cheese

- Dinner: Grilled shrimp with zucchini noodles and a lemon garlic sauce

Thursday:

- Breakfast: Poached eggs with whole-grain toast and sliced tomatoes

- Snack: Fresh berries

- Lunch: Quinoa salad with cucumber, cherry tomatoes, and feta cheese

- Snack: Sugar-free gelatin

- Dinner: Baked chicken with roasted sweet potatoes and green beans

Friday:

- Breakfast: Greek yogurt parfait with granola and sliced strawberries

- Snack: Rice cakes with avocado spread

- Lunch: Grilled vegetable and tofu kebabs

- Snack: Watermelon cubes

- Dinner: Baked cod with steamed Brussels sprouts and wild rice

Saturday:

- Breakfast: Veggie omelet with bell peppers and onions

- Snack: Mixed nuts

- Lunch: Spinach and feta stuffed chicken breast

- Snack: Sliced pear with cottage cheese

- Dinner: Turkey chili with a side of sautéed spinach

Sunday:

- Breakfast: Whole-grain pancakes with sugar-free syrup and blueberries

- Snack: Rice crackers with guacamole

- Lunch: Baked halibut with a side of green salad

- Snack: Melon cubes

- Dinner: Vegetable stir-fry with tofu and brown rice

Grocery Shopping for Diabetes and Kidney-friendly Foods

Grocery shopping for diabetes and kidney-friendly foods is crucial to maintain a healthy diet and manage both conditions effectively. Here's a comprehensive guide to help you make informed choices:

1. Fresh Produce: Opt for low-sugar fruits and non-starchy vegetables, such as berries, apples, broccoli, and spinach. These are rich in essential nutrients and fiber, promoting better blood sugar control and kidney health.

2. Whole Grains: Choose whole grains like quinoa, brown rice, and whole wheat instead of refined grains. Whole grains have a lower glycemic index, which helps regulate blood sugar levels and provides more nutrients.

3. Lean Proteins: Include lean protein sources like skinless poultry, fish, tofu, and legumes. These foods are low in fat and promote better kidney function.

4. Dairy and Alternatives: Opt for low-fat or fat-free dairy products, or non-dairy alternatives like almond milk. Check labels for added sugars and avoid them when possible.

5. Healthy Fats: Select unsaturated fats like olive oil, avocados, and nuts. Limit saturated and trans fats, as they can worsen heart health, which is often a concern for people with diabetes and kidney issues.

6. Limit Sodium: Choose low-sodium or no-added-salt options to support kidney health and manage blood pressure. Be mindful of canned and processed foods, as they often contain high sodium levels.

7. Read Food Labels: Pay attention to the nutritional information on labels. Look for foods with lower carbohydrate and sugar content, as well as reduced sodium and phosphorus levels.

8. Snack Wisely: Opt for snacks like raw veggies, nuts, and seeds rather than sugary or salty options. This helps maintain stable blood sugar and kidney function.

9. Fluid Intake: For those with kidney issues, monitor fluid intake and choose beverages wisely. Water is the best choice, but herbal teas and diluted fruit juices can be consumed in moderation.

10. Portion Control: Keep portions in check to manage blood sugar and avoid overburdening the kidneys. Smaller, balanced meals throughout the day can be more beneficial.

11. Cautious with Sweets: If you have diabetes, limit your intake of sugary treats, and opt for sugar-free alternatives or natural sweeteners in moderation.

By following these guidelines, you can make healthier choices during grocery shopping, supporting both your diabetes management and kidney health.

Batch Cooking and Freezing Meals

Batch cooking and freezing meals can be a valuable strategy for individuals with diabetes and kidney-friendly dietary needs. This approach not only saves time and effort but also promotes healthier eating habits by providing well-balanced and portion-controlled meals.

Here's a comprehensive note on how to effectively batch cook and freeze meals tailored to the specific requirements of diabetes and kidney-friendly diets:

1. Planning and Recipe Selection:

a. Before starting, consult with a registered dietitian or healthcare professional to understand your specific dietary needs and restrictions related to diabetes and kidney health.

b. Choose recipes that are low in sodium, sugar, and unhealthy fats, and focus on nutrient-dense ingredients like lean proteins, whole grains, and fresh vegetables.

2. Grocery Shopping:

a. Make a detailed grocery list based on your selected recipes to ensure you have all the necessary ingredients.

b. Opt for fresh produce and high-quality proteins, and read labels to avoid hidden sugars, excessive sodium, and phosphorus-containing additives.

3. Meal Preparation:

a. Set aside a designated day for batch cooking to streamline the process and maximize efficiency.

b. Prepare larger quantities of your selected recipes, portion them appropriately, and use food-safe containers suitable for freezing.

4. Portion Control and Labeling:

a. Divide the batch-cooked meals into individual portions to prevent overeating and aid in monitoring carbohydrate and nutrient intake.

b. Label each container with the meal name, date of preparation, and reheating instructions for easy identification later.

5. Freezing Guidelines:

a. Allow hot meals to cool slightly before freezing to avoid condensation, which can lead to freezer burn.

b. Use airtight containers or resealable freezer bags to protect the food from freezer odors and maintain freshness.

c. Keep a record of the meals in the freezer, including their expiration dates, to ensure you consume them within a safe time frame.

6. Meal Reheating and Safety:

a. Thaw frozen meals in the refrigerator overnight to ensure even thawing and reduce the risk of bacterial growth.

b. Reheat meals thoroughly to an internal temperature of 165°F (74°C) to eliminate any potential bacteria and ensure they are safe to eat.

c. Avoid reheating meals more than once to maintain their nutritional value and prevent foodborne illnesses.

7. Variety and Balance:

a. Aim for a diverse selection of batch-cooked meals to avoid monotony and keep the eating experience enjoyable.

b. Strive for a balance of macronutrients and limit high-phosphorus ingredients, such as dairy products, nuts, and seeds, to support kidney health.

8. Hydration and Snacking:

a. Stay well-hydrated by drinking plenty of water throughout the day, as proper hydration is vital for kidney function and overall health.

b. Choose kidney-friendly snacks, such as fresh fruits, vegetables, and low-sodium nuts, to complement your batch-cooked meals.

Remember, while batch cooking and freezing can be a convenient solution for managing diabetes and kidney-friendly diets, it's essential to continue working closely with your healthcare team to ensure your dietary plan aligns with your specific health needs and goals.

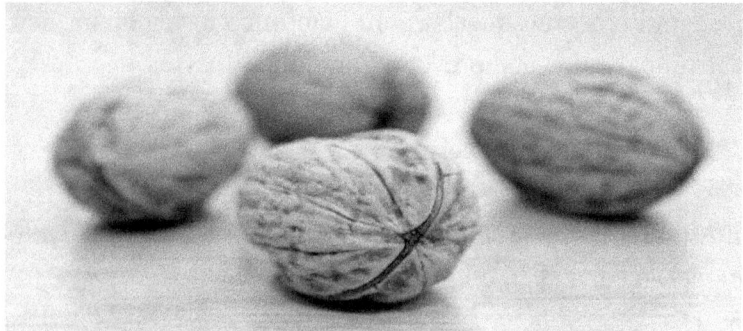

Walnuts

CHAPTER 10

Conclusion

The Diabetes Renal Diet plays a crucial role in managing the complex relationship between diabetes and renal health. With an increasing prevalence of both conditions globally, it has become imperative to adopt dietary strategies that promote blood sugar control while safeguarding kidney function.

The carefully structured Diabetes Renal Diet focuses on controlling carbohydrate intake to manage blood glucose levels, reducing sodium and protein to alleviate the burden on the kidneys, and encouraging the consumption of nutrient-rich, whole foods to support overall health. Additionally, adequate hydration and portion control play pivotal roles in maintaining optimal renal function.

By following this specialized diet, individuals with diabetes and renal complications can significantly improve their quality of life, slow the progression of kidney disease, and reduce the risk of related complications.

Nevertheless, it is essential to consult with healthcare professionals and registered dietitians to tailor the Diabetes Renal Diet to individual needs and ensure its effectiveness and safety in achieving the best possible outcomes.

Dietary management, along with medical care and lifestyle modifications, can be a powerful tool in the battle against diabetes and renal complications.

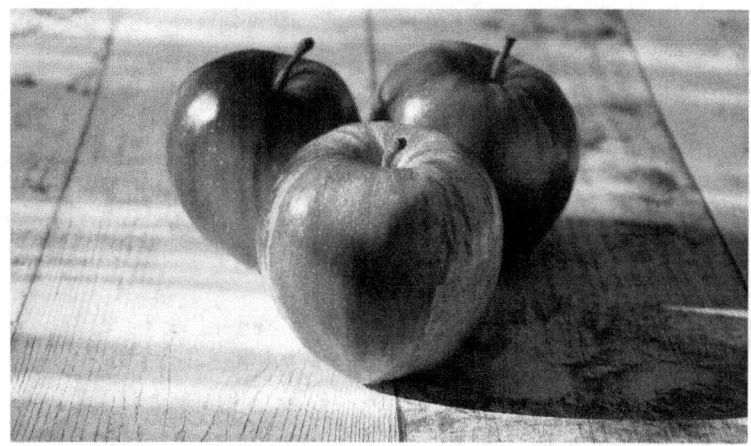

Red Apples

www.ingramcontent.com/pod-product-compliance
Lightning Source LLC
Chambersburg PA
CBHW062324290526
45794CB00005B/1895

* 9 7 9 8 8 5 6 8 8 8 3 8 5 *